WEIGHT WATCHERS DIET BOOK 2023

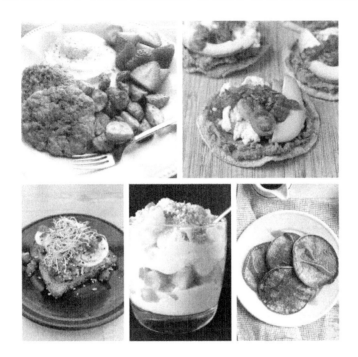

Tasty Recipes with information on Calories, Carbohydrates, Protein, Fats, Sugar, Iron, Calcium, Potassium, Sodium, and Vitamin D

CONTENTS

Publisher's Note

INTRODUCTION

Welcome to the Weight Watchers Diet Book 2023, a comprehensive guide to healthy eating and weight management. Whether you are looking to lose weight, maintain a healthy weight, or simply adopt a healthier lifestyle, this book has everything you need to achieve your goals.

At the heart of the Weight Watchers Diet is the SmartPoints system, which assigns a point value to every food based on its nutritional value including homemade drinks for diet. This system makes it easy to make healthy choices and stay on track with your goals. The SmartPoints system encourages you to eat a variety of nutrient-dense foods, including fruits, vegetables, lean proteins, and whole grains, while still allowing for the occasional treat.

In this book, you will find a variety of recipes, meal plans, and tips to help you stay on track and make healthy choices. Whether you are cooking for one or feeding a family, there are recipes to suit every taste and dietary need, you will have all the resources you need to stay motivated and succeed.

So whether you are just starting out on your weight loss journey or are looking for new ways to maintain a healthy lifestyle, the Weight Watchers Diet Book 2023 is the perfect guide to help you achieve your goals. Let's get started!

CHAPTER ONE

WEIGHT WATCHERS DIET FOOD RECIPES

Grilled salmon with roasted vegetables

Ingredients:

4 salmon fillets (about 6 ounces each)

1 tablespoon olive oil

1 teaspoon dried thyme

Salt and pepper, to taste

2 medium zucchini, sliced

1 medium red onion, sliced

1 red bell pepper, sliced

1 tablespoon balsamic vinegar

2 teaspoons honey

Directions:

- Preheat the oven to 400°F (200°C).

- In a bowl, mix together the olive oil, thyme, salt, and pepper. Brush the salmon fillets with the mixture and set aside.

- In a separate bowl, toss together the zucchini, red onion, and red bell pepper with the balsamic vinegar and honey.

- Spread the vegetables out in a single layer on a baking sheet. Roast in the preheated oven for 20-25 minutes, until tender and lightly browned.

- While the vegetables are roasting, heat a grill pan over medium-high heat. Add the salmon fillets and cook for 3-4 minutes on each side, until cooked through.

- Serve the grilled salmon with the roasted vegetables on the side.

This recipe makes 4 servings. Each serving contains approximately 300 calories, 25 grams of protein, and 12 grams of fat. It's a healthy and satisfying meal that is perfect for anyone following a weight watchers diet.

Shrimp and vegetable stir-fry with brown rice

Ingredients:

1 pound large shrimp, peeled and deveined

2 tablespoons cornstarch

1 tablespoon vegetable oil

1 tablespoon minced garlic

1 tablespoon minced ginger

1 small red onion, sliced

1 red bell pepper, sliced

1 cup sliced carrots

1 cup broccoli florets

1/2 cup sliced water chestnuts

1/4 cup low-sodium soy sauce

2 tablespoons oyster sauce

2 tablespoons rice vinegar

1 tablespoon honey

4 cups cooked brown rice

Directions:

- In a small bowl, toss the shrimp with cornstarch until coated.

- Heat the vegetable oil in a large skillet or wok over medium-high heat. Add the garlic and ginger and stir-fry for 30 seconds.

- Add the onion, bell pepper, carrots, broccoli, and water chestnuts and stir-fry for 3-4 minutes, until the vegetables are tender-crisp.

- Add the shrimp to the skillet and stir-fry for 2-3 minutes, until the shrimp are pink and cooked through.

- In a small bowl, whisk together the soy sauce, oyster sauce, rice vinegar, and honey. Pour the sauce over the shrimp and vegetables and stir to coat.

- Serve the shrimp and vegetable stir-fry over the cooked brown rice.

This recipe makes 4 servings. Each serving contains approximately 400 calories, 25 grams of protein, and 7 grams of fat. It's a healthy and flavorful meal that is perfect for anyone following a weight watchers diet.

Chicken and vegetable kebabs with tzatziki sauce

Ingredients:

4 boneless, skinless chicken breasts, cut into cubes

2 medium bell peppers, cut into chunks

1 medium red onion, cut into chunks

1 zucchini, cut into chunks

1 tbsp olive oil

Salt and pepper, to taste

Skewers (if using wooden skewers, soak them in water for 30 minutes before using)

For tzatziki sauce:

1 cup plain Greek yogurt

1/2 cup grated cucumber, squeezed to remove excess water

1 garlic clove, minced

1 tbsp lemon juice

Salt and pepper, to taste

Directions:

- Preheat the grill to medium-high heat.

- Thread the chicken and vegetables onto skewers, alternating between chicken, peppers, onion, and zucchini. Brush with olive oil and season with salt and pepper.

- Grill the kebabs for 10-12 minutes, turning occasionally, until the chicken is cooked through.

- Meanwhile, prepare the tzatziki sauce by combining the yogurt, cucumber, garlic, lemon juice, salt, and pepper in a small bowl.

- Serve the kebabs hot with tzatziki sauce on the side.

This recipe serves 4 and each serving contains approximately 7 SmartPoints on the Weight Watchers diet. Enjoy!

Slow-cooker vegetable soup

Ingredients:

1 large onion, diced

2 cloves garlic, minced

3 carrots, peeled and diced

3 stalks celery, diced

1 can diced tomatoes, drained

6 cups low-sodium vegetable broth

1 teaspoon dried thyme

1 teaspoon dried rosemary

1 teaspoon dried oregano

1 bay leaf

2 cups chopped kale or spinach

Salt and pepper, to taste

Instructions:

- In a slow cooker, add the onion, garlic, carrots, celery, and diced tomatoes.

- Pour in the vegetable broth and stir to combine.

- Add the thyme, rosemary, oregano, bay leaf, and a pinch of salt and pepper.

- Cover and cook on low for 6-8 hours or high for 3-4 hours.

- Stir in the chopped kale or spinach during the last 30 minutes of cooking.

- Remove the bay leaf and season with additional salt and pepper, if needed.

- Serve hot and enjoy!

This recipe makes 6-8 servings and is perfect for meal prep or freezing for later. Each serving is low in calories and high in fiber, making it a great option for weight watchers.

Baked chicken with mushroom sauce

Ingredients:

4 boneless, skinless chicken breasts

2 tbsp olive oil

1 tbsp garlic powder

1 tbsp onion powder

1 tbsp paprika

Salt and pepper, to taste

1 cup sliced mushrooms

1 tbsp butter

2 tbsp all-purpose flour

1 cup low-sodium chicken broth

1/2 cup low-fat milk

Instructions:

- Preheat the oven to 375°F (190°C).

- In a small bowl, mix together olive oil, garlic powder, onion powder, paprika, salt, and pepper.
- Place the chicken breasts in a baking dish and rub the seasoning mixture all over them.

- Bake for 25-30 minutes, or until the chicken is cooked through.

- While the chicken is cooking, prepare the mushroom sauce. Heat the butter in a saucepan over medium heat.

- Add the sliced mushrooms and sauté for 3-4 minutes, or until they are soft.

- Sprinkle the flour over the mushrooms and stir until it's fully coated.

- Gradually pour in the chicken broth and milk, whisking constantly to prevent lumps.

- Bring the sauce to a simmer and cook for 5-7 minutes, or until it thickens and becomes creamy.

- Remove the chicken from the oven and let it rest for a few minutes.

- Spoon the mushroom sauce over the chicken breasts and serve.

This recipe makes 4 servings and each serving contains approximately 300 calories. It's a great option for a healthy and satisfying dinner for weight watchers.

Broiled cod with asparagus and cherry tomatoes

Ingredients:

4 4-oz cod fillets

1 lb asparagus, trimmed

1 pint cherry tomatoes, halved

2 cloves garlic, minced

2 tbsp olive oil

Salt and pepper, to taste

Instructions:

- Preheat the broiler too high.

- Arrange the asparagus and cherry tomatoes on a baking sheet. Drizzle with 1 tablespoon of olive oil and season with salt and pepper.

- Broil the asparagus and tomatoes for 5-7 minutes, or until the asparagus is tender and the tomatoes are slightly charred.

- While the asparagus and tomatoes are cooking, season the cod fillets with salt and pepper.

- In a separate pan, heat the remaining tablespoon of olive oil over medium heat. Add the minced garlic and cook for 1-2 minutes, or until fragrant.

- Add the cod fillets to the pan and cook for 4-5 minutes per side, or until cooked through.

- Serve the cod fillets with the roasted asparagus and cherry tomatoes.

This recipe serves 4 and each serving contains approximately 236 calories, making it a great choice for a weight watchers diet.

Grilled flank steak with roasted vegetables

Ingredients:

1 pound flank steak

2 tablespoons olive oil

2 teaspoons garlic powder

2 teaspoons onion powder

1 teaspoon paprika

1/2 teaspoon salt

1/4 teaspoon black pepper

1 red bell pepper, sliced

1 yellow bell pepper, sliced

1 zucchini, sliced

1 red onion, sliced

Cooking spray

Instructions:

- Preheat your oven to 400°F.

- Combine the garlic powder, onion powder, paprika, salt, and black pepper in a small bowl.

- Rub the spice mixture all over the flank steak.

- Heat a grill pan over medium-high heat. Add the flank steak and cook for 4-5 minutes per side, or until it reaches your desired level of doneness.

- While the steak is cooking, prepare the vegetables. Toss the sliced peppers, zucchini, and red onion with 2 tablespoons of olive oil and spread them out on a baking sheet. Spray the vegetables with cooking spray.

- Roast the vegetables in the preheated oven for 15-20 minutes, or until they are tender and slightly browned.

- Let the steak rest for a few minutes before slicing it thinly against the grain.

- Serve the sliced steak with the roasted vegetables on the side.

This recipe serves 4 and each serving is approximately 8 WW SmartPoints (calculated using the WW recipe builder).

Turkey and quinoa stuffed peppers

Ingredients:

4 large bell peppers (any color)

1 pound ground turkey

1/2 cup quinoa

1 onion, chopped

2 cloves garlic, minced

1 can diced tomatoes

1 tablespoon tomato paste

1 teaspoon dried basil

1 teaspoon dried oregano

1/2 teaspoon salt

1/4 teaspoon black pepper

1 cup water

1/2 cup shredded low-fat cheddar cheese

Cooking spray

Instructions:

- Preheat the oven to 375°F.

- Cut off the tops of the bell peppers and remove the seeds and membranes. Rinse and set aside.

- In a large skillet, cook the ground turkey over medium-high heat until browned. Drain any excess fat.

- Add the chopped onion and minced garlic to the skillet and cook until the onion is translucent.

- Add the quinoa, diced tomatoes, tomato paste, basil, oregano, salt, and black pepper to the skillet. Stir to combine.

- Add 1 cup of water and bring the mixture to a boil. Reduce heat to low and simmer for 20-25 minutes, or until the quinoa is cooked through.

- Spray a baking dish with cooking spray. Stuff each bell pepper with the turkey and quinoa mixture and place in the baking dish.

- Cover the baking dish with aluminum foil and bake for 30 minutes.

- Remove the aluminum foil, sprinkle the shredded cheese over the stuffed peppers, and bake for an additional 10-15 minutes, or until the cheese is melted and bubbly.

- Let the stuffed peppers cool for a few minutes before serving.

This recipe makes 4 servings, each stuffed pepper is approximately 6 WW SmartPoints. Enjoy!

Roasted vegetable and quinoa salad

Ingredients:

1 cup quinoa

2 cups water

1 red onion, sliced

2 bell peppers, sliced

1 zucchini, sliced

1 eggplant, sliced

2 tablespoons olive oil

2 cloves garlic, minced

Salt and pepper to taste

1/4 cup fresh parsley, chopped

1/4 cup fresh basil, chopped

2 tablespoons balsamic vinegar

Directions:

- Preheat the oven to 400°F (200°C).

- Rinse the quinoa in a fine mesh strainer under cold water. Add the quinoa and water to a medium saucepan and bring to a boil over high heat. Reduce the heat to low, cover, and simmer for 15-20 minutes or until the water is absorbed and the quinoa is cooked through. Set aside.

- In a large bowl, toss the sliced red onion, bell peppers, zucchini, and eggplant with olive oil, garlic, salt, and pepper. Spread the vegetables out on a baking sheet and roast for 20-25 minutes or until tender and golden brown. Let cool for 5 minutes.

- In a large bowl, combine the cooked quinoa, roasted vegetables, fresh parsley, and basil. Toss gently to combine.

- Drizzle the balsamic vinegar over the salad and toss again.

- Serve immediately or refrigerate until ready to serve.

This recipe makes 4 servings and each serving is 7 Weight Watchers SmartPoints. Enjoy!

Grilled pork chops with roasted sweet potatoes

Ingredients:

4 bone-in pork chops

2 tablespoons olive oil

2 cloves garlic, minced

1 tablespoon chopped fresh rosemary

Salt and pepper to taste

2 large sweet potatoes, peeled and cut into cubes

1 tablespoon honey

1 tablespoon balsamic vinegar

Directions:

- Preheat a grill to medium-high heat.

- In a small bowl, mix together the olive oil, garlic, rosemary, salt, and pepper. Brush the mixture over both sides of the pork chops.

- Grill the pork chops for 4-5 minutes per side, or until cooked through. Remove from the grill and let rest for 5 minutes.

- While the pork chops are grilling, preheat the oven to 400°F (200°C).

- Place the sweet potato cubes in a large bowl. Drizzle with olive oil and sprinkle with salt and pepper. Toss to coat.

- Spread the sweet potatoes out on a baking sheet and roast for 20-25 minutes or until tender and golden brown.

- In a small bowl, whisk together the honey and balsamic vinegar.

- Serve the pork chops with the roasted sweet potatoes, drizzled with the honey-balsamic mixture.

Baked salmon with roasted Brussels sprouts

Ingredients:
4 (4-ounce) salmon fillets
1 lb Brussels sprouts, trimmed and halved
2 tbsp olive oil
1/2 tsp salt
1/4 tsp black pepper

1/4 tsp garlic powder

1/4 tsp onion powder

1/4 tsp paprika

1 lemon, cut into wedges

Directions:

- Preheat the oven to 400°F.

- In a large bowl, toss the Brussels sprouts with 1 tablespoon of olive oil, salt, and black pepper. Spread them out in a single layer on a baking sheet.

- Roast the Brussels sprouts for 20-25 minutes, or until tender and lightly browned.

- While the Brussels sprouts are roasting, season the salmon fillets with garlic powder, onion powder, paprika, salt, and black pepper. Drizzle them with the remaining tablespoon of olive oil.

- Place the salmon fillets on another baking sheet lined with parchment paper, skin-side down.

- Bake for 12-15 minutes, or until the salmon is cooked through and flakes easily with a fork.

- Serve the salmon and roasted Brussels sprouts with lemon wedges on the side for squeezing over the top.

This recipe is a healthy and delicious way to enjoy salmon and Brussels sprouts while on a Weight Watchers diet. Each serving contains approximately 6 Weight Watchers SmartPoints.

Slow-cooker chicken chili

Ingredients:

1 pound boneless, skinless chicken breasts, cubed

1 can (15 ounces) black beans, rinsed and drained

1 can (15 ounces) kidney beans, rinsed and drained

1 can (15 ounces) corn, drained

1 can (15 ounces) diced tomatoes

1 can (4 ounces) diced green chilies

1 onion, chopped

1 red bell pepper, chopped

2 cloves garlic, minced

1 tablespoon chili powder

1 teaspoon cumin

1/2 teaspoon salt

1/2 teaspoon black pepper

1 cup low-sodium chicken broth

Instructions:

- Add the chicken, beans, corn, diced tomatoes, green chilies, onion, bell pepper, garlic, chili powder, cumin, salt, and black pepper to a 6-quart slow cooker.

- Stir everything together until well combined.

- Pour in the chicken broth and stir again.

- Cover the slow cooker and cook on low for 6 to 8 hours or on high for 3 to 4 hours.

- When the chicken is cooked through and the vegetables are tender, taste the chili and adjust the seasoning as needed.

- Serve hot, topped with your favorite garnishes, such as shredded cheese, sour cream, or chopped fresh cilantro.

This recipe makes about 8 servings, each with approximately 300 calories and 5 WW SmartPoints per serving. Enjoy!

Baked chicken parmesan

Ingredients:
4 boneless, skinless chicken breasts (about 1.5 lbs)
1/2 cup all-purpose flour
1/2 tsp salt
1/4 tsp black pepper
2 large eggs

1 cup seasoned breadcrumbs

1/2 cup grated Parmesan cheese

1/2 cup reduced-fat shredded mozzarella cheese

2 cups marinara sauce

Cooking spray

Instructions:

- Preheat the oven to 400°F.

- In a shallow dish, combine flour, salt, and black pepper.

- In another shallow dish, whisk together eggs.

- In a third shallow dish, combine breadcrumbs and Parmesan cheese.

- Dredge each chicken breast in the flour mixture, shaking off any excess. Dip in egg mixture, then coat in breadcrumb mixture.

- Place chicken breasts on a baking sheet coated with cooking spray.

- Bake for 20 minutes, then remove from oven and spoon 1/4 cup marinara sauce over each chicken breast.

- Top each chicken breast with 2 tablespoons of shredded mozzarella cheese.

- Return to the oven and bake for an additional 10-15 minutes, or until chicken is cooked through and cheese is melted and bubbly.

- Serve hot, with additional marinara sauce and Parmesan cheese on the side, if desired.

This recipe makes 4 servings, with each serving containing approximately 365 calories, 12g fat, 26g carbohydrates, 2g fiber, and 40g protein. Enjoy!

Grilled shrimp and vegetable skewers with pineapple salsa

Ingredients:

For the skewers:
1 lb. large shrimp, peeled and deveined
1 medium red bell pepper, cut into 1-inch pieces
1 medium yellow bell pepper, cut into 1-inch pieces
1 medium zucchini, cut into 1/2-inch rounds
1 medium red onion, cut into 1-inch pieces
1 tablespoon olive oil
Salt and black pepper to taste

For the pineapple salsa:
1 cup diced pineapple
1/4 cup finely chopped red onion
1/4 cup finely chopped fresh cilantro

1 tablespoon fresh lime juice
Salt and black pepper to taste

Instructions:

- Preheat the grill to medium-high heat.

- In a large bowl, combine the shrimp, bell peppers, zucchini, red onion, olive oil, salt, and black pepper. Toss well to coat.

- Thread the shrimp and vegetables onto skewers, alternating the different ingredients.

- Grill the skewers for 4-5 minutes per side, until the shrimp are pink and cooked through.

- While the skewers are grilling, make the pineapple salsa by combining the diced pineapple, red onion, cilantro, lime juice, salt, and black pepper in a small bowl. Mix well.

- Serve the skewers hot, topped with the pineapple salsa.

This recipe makes 4 servings, and each serving has around 6 Weight Watchers SmartPoints, depending on the size of the shrimp and the amount of olive oil used. Enjoy!

Roasted turkey breast with green beans and mashed sweet potatoes

Ingredients:

For the turkey:
1 lb. boneless turkey breast

1 tablespoon olive oil

1 teaspoon dried thyme

1 teaspoon dried rosemary

Salt and black pepper to taste

For the green beans:
1 lb. fresh green beans, trimmed

1 tablespoon olive oil

2 garlic cloves, minced

Salt and black pepper to taste

For the mashed sweet potatoes:
2 lbs. sweet potatoes, peeled and cut into 1-inch cubes

1/4 cup low-fat milk

1 tablespoon butter

Salt and black pepper to taste

Instructions:

- Preheat the oven to 375°F.

- Rub the turkey breast with the olive oil and sprinkle with thyme, rosemary, salt, and black pepper. Place the turkey in a roasting pan and roast for 45-50 minutes, or until the internal temperature reaches 165°F.

- While the turkey is roasting, prepare the green beans. In a large bowl, toss the green beans with the olive oil, garlic, salt, and black pepper. Spread the green beans out on a baking sheet and roast for 15-20 minutes, or until tender and slightly browned.

- Boil the sweet potato cubes in a large pot of salted water until tender, about 15 minutes. Drain and mash the sweet potatoes with the milk, butter, salt, and black pepper.

- Serve the roasted turkey breast with the green beans and mashed sweet potatoes.

This recipe makes 4 servings, and each serving has around 8-9 Weight Watchers SmartPoints, depending on the size of the turkey breast and the amount of butter used in the sweet potatoes. Enjoy!

Chicken and vegetable curry

Ingredients:
1 lb. boneless, skinless chicken breasts, cut into bite-sized pieces
1 tablespoon olive oil
1 large onion, chopped

2 garlic cloves, minced

1 tablespoon grated fresh ginger

2 tablespoons curry powder

1 teaspoon ground cumin

1/2 teaspoon ground coriander

1/4 teaspoon ground cinnamon

1/4 teaspoon cayenne pepper

1 can (14.5 oz) diced tomatoes, undrained

1 can (13.5 oz) light coconut milk

1 large sweet potato, peeled and cut into bite-sized pieces

1 red bell pepper, cut into bite-sized pieces

1 green bell pepper, cut into bite-sized pieces

Salt and black pepper to taste

1/4 cup chopped fresh cilantro, for garnish

Cooked brown rice, for serving

Instructions:

- Heat the olive oil in a large saucepan or Dutch oven over medium-high heat. Add the chicken and cook until browned on all sides, about 5 minutes. Remove the chicken from the pan and set aside.

- Add the onion, garlic, and ginger to the same pan and cook until softened, about 3 minutes.

- Add the curry powder, cumin, coriander, cinnamon, and cayenne pepper to the pan and stir well. Cook for 1 minute, stirring constantly.

- Add the diced tomatoes with their juice, coconut milk, sweet potato, and bell peppers to the pan. Bring to a simmer and cook for 10-15 minutes, or until the sweet potato is tender and the sauce has thickened.

- Add the cooked chicken to the pan and stir well. Season with salt and black pepper to taste.

- Serve the chicken and vegetable curry hot, garnished with chopped cilantro and with brown rice on the side.

This recipe makes 4 servings, and each serving has around 7-8 Weight Watchers SmartPoints, depending on the amount of rice used. Enjoy!

Roasted vegetable and chicken quinoa bowl

Ingredients:

1 cup quinoa

2 cups water

1 large chicken breast, sliced

1 small eggplant, diced

1 red bell pepper, diced

1 zucchini, diced

1 onion, diced

2 cloves garlic, minced

1 tablespoon olive oil

Salt and pepper to taste

For the dressing:

2 tablespoons balsamic vinegar

1 tablespoon Dijon mustard

1 tablespoon honey

1/4 cup olive oil

Directions:

- Preheat the oven to 400 degrees F.

- In a pot, combine quinoa and water. Bring to a boil, reduce heat, and simmer for about 20 minutes or until the water is absorbed and the quinoa is cooked through.

- While the quinoa is cooking, prepare the vegetables. Toss the eggplant, red bell pepper, zucchini, onion, and garlic with olive oil, salt, and pepper. Spread the vegetables on a baking sheet and roast in the preheated oven for 20-25 minutes or until they are tender and slightly browned.

- In a pan, cook the chicken slices until browned and cooked through.

- In a small bowl, whisk together the balsamic vinegar, Dijon mustard, honey, and olive oil to make the dressing.

- To assemble the bowl, place cooked quinoa in a bowl, then top with the roasted vegetables and chicken. Drizzle with the dressing and serve.

This recipe should make about 4 servings, and each serving contains approximately:

383 calories
14g fat
42g carbohydrates
26g protein
Note: These nutritional values are approximate and may vary depending on the exact ingredients used.

Grilled vegetable and tofu skewers

Ingredients:
14 oz. extra firm tofu, drained and cut into 1-inch cubes
1 large red onion, cut into 1-inch pieces
2 large bell peppers (red, yellow, or green), seeded and cut into 1-inch pieces
2 medium zucchinis, cut into 1/2-inch rounds
2 tbsp. olive oil

1 tbsp. balsamic vinegar

1 tbsp. chopped fresh basil

1 tsp. dried oregano

Salt and pepper, to taste

Skewers (if using wooden skewers, soak them in water for at least 30 minutes)

Instructions:

- Preheat the grill to medium-high heat.

- Thread tofu, red onion, bell peppers, and zucchinis onto skewers.

- In a small bowl, whisk together olive oil, balsamic vinegar, basil, oregano, salt, and pepper.

- Brush the skewers with the olive oil mixture.
- Place the skewers on the grill and cook for 5-7 minutes per side, or until the vegetables are tender and lightly charred.

- Serve hot and enjoy!

This recipe serves 4 and contains approximately 220 calories per serving. It is a great source of protein and fiber, and is also low in fat and carbohydrates. Enjoy!

Slow-cooker turkey and vegetable soup

Ingredients:

1 pound of turkey breast, cooked and shredded

4 cups of low-sodium chicken broth

1 can (14.5 oz) of diced tomatoes

2 cups of mixed vegetables (carrots, celery, onion, zucchini, etc.)

1 cup of frozen corn

1 tsp of dried thyme

1 tsp of dried oregano

1 tsp of garlic powder

Salt and pepper to taste

Instructions:

- In a slow cooker, add the cooked and shredded turkey breast, chicken broth, diced tomatoes, mixed vegetables, and frozen corn.

- Stir in the dried thyme, dried oregano, garlic powder, salt, and pepper.

- Cook on low for 6-8 hours or on high for 3-4 hours.

- Serve hot and enjoy!

Weight Watchers Points:

This recipe makes 6 servings, and each serving is approximately 1 1/2 cups. Each serving is 1 point on the Weight Watchers diet.

Baked tilapia with roasted broccoli

Ingredients:

4 tilapia fillets (4-6 ounces each)

1 head of broccoli, cut into florets

2 tablespoons olive oil

2 teaspoons lemon zest

2 tablespoons lemon juice

2 garlic cloves, minced

1/2 teaspoon salt

1/4 teaspoon black pepper

Instructions:

- Preheat the oven to 400°F (200°C).

- In a small bowl, whisk together the olive oil, lemon zest, lemon juice, garlic, salt, and pepper.

- Place the tilapia fillets in a baking dish and pour the marinade over them. Let them marinate for 15 minutes.

- Meanwhile, place the broccoli florets on a baking sheet and toss with a tablespoon of olive oil, salt, and pepper.

- Place the baking sheet in the oven and roast the broccoli for 15-20 minutes, or until tender and slightly browned.

- After the tilapia has finished marinating, place the baking dish in the oven and bake for 10-12 minutes, or until the fish is cooked through and flakes easily with a fork.

- Serve the tilapia with the roasted broccoli on the side.

This recipe makes 4 servings, with each serving containing approximately 220 calories, 8 grams of fat, and 0 grams of carbohydrates (source: Weight Watchers). Enjoy!

Pork tenderloin with roasted vegetables

Ingredients:
1 lb. pork tenderloin
2 tablespoons olive oil
Salt and pepper, to taste
1 teaspoon dried thyme
1 teaspoon garlic powder
1/2 teaspoon onion powder
1 red bell pepper, sliced
1 yellow bell pepper, sliced
1 medium zucchini, sliced

1 medium onion, sliced
1 tablespoon balsamic vinegar

Instructions:

- Preheat the oven to 400 degrees F.

- In a small bowl, mix together the thyme, garlic powder, onion powder, salt, and pepper.

- Rub the spice mixture all over the pork tenderloin.

- Heat 1 tablespoon of olive oil in a large oven-safe skillet over medium-high heat.

- Add the pork tenderloin to the skillet and sear for 2-3 minutes on each side, until browned.

- Transfer the skillet to the oven and roast for 15-20 minutes, or until the internal temperature of the pork reaches 145 degrees F.

- Meanwhile, in a large bowl, combine the sliced bell peppers, zucchini, and onion.

- Drizzle with the remaining tablespoon of olive oil and toss to coat.

- Spread the vegetables out on a large baking sheet in a single layer.

- Roast the vegetables in the preheated oven for 20-25 minutes, or until tender and lightly browned.

- Remove the pork tenderloin from the skillet and let it rest for 5-10 minutes before slicing.

- Drizzle the roasted vegetables with balsamic vinegar and serve alongside the sliced pork tenderloin.

Note: The Weight Watchers SmartPoints for this recipe will depend on the specific ingredients you use, so be sure to calculate the SmartPoints based on the brands and amounts you choose.

Chicken and vegetable stir-fry with soba noodles

Ingredients:

8 oz soba noodles

2 tbsp vegetable oil

1 lb boneless, skinless chicken breasts, cut into bite-sized pieces

1 red bell pepper, sliced

1 yellow bell pepper, sliced

1 zucchini, sliced

1 onion, sliced

3 garlic cloves, minced

1/4 cup low-sodium soy sauce

1 tbsp honey

1 tbsp cornstarch

1/4 cup water

Salt and pepper to taste

Chopped green onions, for garnish

Instructions:

- Cook the soba noodles according to package instructions. Drain and set aside.

- In a large skillet or wok, heat 1 tbsp of the vegetable oil over medium-high heat.

- Add the chicken and stir-fry for about 5-7 minutes until browned and cooked through. Remove the chicken from the skillet and set aside.

- In the same skillet, heat the remaining 1 tbsp of vegetable oil over medium-high heat.

- Add the bell peppers, zucchini, onion, and garlic. Stir-fry for about 3-5 minutes until the vegetables are crisp-tender.

- In a small bowl, whisk together the soy sauce, honey, cornstarch, and water.

- Add the chicken back to the skillet with the vegetables.

- Pour the soy sauce mixture over the chicken and vegetables and stir to coat.

- Cook for an additional 1-2 minutes until the sauce has thickened.

- Season with salt and pepper to taste.

- Serve the chicken and vegetable stir-fry over the cooked soba noodles.

- Garnish with chopped green onions before serving.

This recipe makes 4 servings, and each serving contains approximately 362 calories, 7g fat, 46g carbohydrates, 28g protein, and 6 WW SmartPoints (Blue, Green, Purple).

Slow-cooker beef and vegetable stew

Ingredients:

1 lb lean beef stew meat, cut into bite-sized pieces

2 tbsp all-purpose flour

Salt and pepper to taste

1 tbsp olive oil

1 onion, chopped

2 cloves garlic, minced

2 cups low-sodium beef broth

2 tbsp tomato paste

2 carrots, chopped

2 stalks celery, chopped

1 lb potatoes, chopped

1 tsp dried thyme

1 bay leaf

Chopped fresh parsley, for garnish

Instructions:

- In a large bowl, toss the beef stew meat with the flour, salt, and pepper until evenly coated.

- Heat the olive oil in a large skillet over medium-high heat.
- Add the beef to the skillet and cook for about 5-7 minutes until browned on all sides. Remove the beef from the skillet and set aside.

- Add the onion and garlic to the skillet and sauté for about 3-5 minutes until the onion is translucent.

- In a slow cooker, combine the beef broth and tomato paste.

- Add the browned beef, sautéed onion and garlic, carrots, celery, potatoes, thyme, and bay leaf to the slow cooker.

- Stir everything together to combine.

- Cover the slow cooker and cook on low for 8-10 hours or on high for 4-6 hours, until the beef and vegetables are tender.

- Remove the bay leaf from the slow cooker.

- Ladle the stew into bowls and garnish with chopped fresh parsley before serving.

This recipe makes 6 servings, and each serving contains approximately 279 calories, 7g fat, 28g carbohydrates, 26g protein, and 4 WW SmartPoints (Blue, Green, Purple).

Grilled vegetable and tofu kebabs with peanut sauce

Ingredients:
1 block of firm tofu, pressed and cut into cubes
1 red bell pepper, seeded and cut into chunks
1 yellow bell pepper, seeded and cut into chunks
1 red onion, cut into chunks
8-10 cherry tomatoes
2 tablespoons olive oil
Salt and pepper, to taste
Wooden skewers

For the peanut sauce:
1/4 cup natural peanut butter
1 tablespoon soy sauce

1 tablespoon honey

1 tablespoon rice vinegar

1/2 teaspoon sesame oil

1/2 teaspoon grated ginger

1 clove garlic, minced

Water, as needed to thin out the sauce

Instructions:

- Preheat your grill to medium-high heat.

- In a large bowl, toss the tofu, red and yellow bell peppers, red onion, cherry tomatoes, olive oil, salt, and pepper together until well coated.

- Thread the vegetables and tofu onto the wooden skewers, alternating between vegetables and tofu.

- Place the skewers on the preheated grill and cook for 8-10 minutes, turning occasionally, until the vegetables are tender and the tofu is lightly charred.

- While the kebabs are cooking, make the peanut sauce. In a small bowl, whisk together the peanut butter, soy sauce, honey, rice vinegar, sesame oil, grated ginger, and minced garlic. Add water to thin out the sauce until it reaches your desired consistency.

- Once the kebabs are done, remove them from the grill and serve with the peanut sauce on the side.

Nutrition information (per serving):
Calories: 237
Fat: 16.1g
Carbohydrates: 14.5g
Fiber: 3.5g
Protein: 12.2g
This recipe makes 4 servings. Enjoy!

Baked chicken and vegetable casserole

Ingredients:
4 boneless, skinless chicken breasts
1 tablespoon olive oil
1 medium onion, chopped
3 garlic cloves, minced
2 medium zucchinis, chopped
1 red bell pepper, chopped
1 yellow bell pepper, chopped
1 teaspoon dried basil
1 teaspoon dried oregano
Salt and pepper, to taste
1 can (14.5 oz) diced tomatoes, drained

1 cup reduced-fat shredded mozzarella cheese
Cooking spray

Instructions:

- Preheat the oven to 375°F (190°C).

- Heat the olive oil in a large skillet over medium-high heat. Add the onion and garlic and sauté until the onion is translucent.

- Add the zucchini, red bell pepper, and yellow bell pepper to the skillet. Season with basil, oregano, salt, and pepper. Sauté until the vegetables are tender, about 10 minutes.
- Add the diced tomatoes to the skillet and stir to combine.

- Cut the chicken breasts into bite-sized pieces and add them to the skillet. Cook until the chicken is no longer pink, about 10 minutes.

- Spray a 9x13-inch baking dish with cooking spray.

- Transfer the chicken and vegetable mixture to the baking dish. Sprinkle the shredded mozzarella cheese on top.

- Bake for 20 minutes or until the cheese is melted and bubbly.

This recipe serves 6 and each serving has approximately 6 SmartPoints on the Weight Watchers diet. Enjoy!

Roasted vegetable and chicken salad

Ingredients:

4 boneless, skinless chicken breasts

1 red bell pepper, sliced

1 yellow bell pepper, sliced

1 small zucchini, sliced

1 small yellow squash, sliced

1 small red onion, sliced

1 tablespoon olive oil

Salt and pepper, to taste

6 cups mixed greens

1/2 cup cherry tomatoes, halved

2 tablespoons balsamic vinegar

2 tablespoons reduced-fat feta cheese

Instructions:

- Preheat the oven to 400°F (200°C).

- Place the chicken breasts on a baking sheet and season with salt and pepper.

- In a separate bowl, toss the sliced peppers, zucchini, yellow squash, and red onion with the olive oil and season with salt and pepper.

- Spread the vegetables on the same baking sheet as the chicken.

- Roast the chicken and vegetables for 20-25 minutes or until the chicken is cooked through and the vegetables are tender.

- Let the chicken and vegetables cool for a few minutes and then slice the chicken into bite-sized pieces.

- Divide the mixed greens between four plates.

- Top the greens with the sliced chicken and roasted vegetables.

- Sprinkle the cherry tomatoes on top of each salad.
- Drizzle the balsamic vinegar over the salads and top with crumbled feta cheese.

This recipe serves 4 and each serving has approximately 4 SmartPoints on the Weight Watchers diet. Enjoy!

Grilled shrimp with zucchini noodles

Ingredients:

1 pound large shrimp, peeled and deveined

1 tablespoon olive oil

2 garlic cloves, minced

1/2 teaspoon salt

1/4 teaspoon black pepper

4 medium zucchinis, spiralized into noodles

1 tablespoon butter

1/4 cup chopped fresh parsley

2 tablespoons grated Parmesan cheese

Instructions:

- Preheat the grill to medium-high heat.

- In a large bowl, combine the shrimp, olive oil, garlic, salt, and pepper. Toss to coat the shrimp.

- Thread the shrimp onto skewers.

- Grill the shrimp for 2-3 minutes per side, or until cooked through.

- While the shrimp is grilling, melt the butter in a large skillet over medium heat.

- Add the zucchini noodles to the skillet and sauté for 2-3 minutes, or until tender.

- Divide the zucchini noodles between four plates.

- Top the zucchini noodles with the grilled shrimp.

- Sprinkle fresh parsley and grated Parmesan cheese over each plate.

This recipe serves 4 and each serving has approximately 3 SmartPoints on the Weight Watchers diet. Enjoy!

Slow-cooker vegetable and lentil soup

Ingredients:
1 tablespoon olive oil
1 medium onion, chopped
2 garlic cloves, minced
2 medium carrots, chopped
2 celery stalks, chopped
1 medium sweet potato, peeled and chopped
1 cup dried green or brown lentils, rinsed and drained
1 can (14.5 oz) diced tomatoes, undrained
4 cups low-sodium vegetable broth
1 teaspoon dried thyme
1 teaspoon dried oregano
Salt and black pepper, to taste
4 cups baby spinach leaves, loosely packed
2 tablespoons fresh lemon juice

Instructions:

- Heat the olive oil in a large skillet over medium heat. Add the onion and garlic and sauté until the onion is translucent.

- Transfer the onion and garlic to a slow cooker.

- Add the chopped carrots, celery, sweet potato, lentils, diced tomatoes, vegetable broth, thyme, oregano, salt, and black pepper to the slow cooker. Stir to combine.

- Cover and cook on low for 6-8 hours or until the lentils and vegetables are tender.

- Stir in the baby spinach leaves and lemon juice. Cover and cook for an additional 5-10 minutes or until the spinach is wilted.

- Taste and adjust the seasoning as needed. Serve hot.

This recipe makes 6 servings and each serving has approximately 4 SmartPoints on the Weight Watchers diet. Enjoy!

Baked sweet potato and black bean chili

Ingredients:

2 large sweet potatoes, peeled and chopped into bite-size pieces

1 tablespoon olive oil

1 onion, chopped

1 red bell pepper, chopped

3 cloves garlic, minced

1 teaspoon ground cumin

1 teaspoon chili powder

1/2 teaspoon paprika

1/4 teaspoon cayenne pepper

1 can (15 oz) black beans, drained and rinsed

1 can (14.5 oz) diced tomatoes, undrained

1/2 cup vegetable broth

Salt and pepper to taste

Optional toppings: chopped fresh cilantro, shredded cheese, sour cream or Greek yogurt

Instructions:

- Preheat the oven to 375°F.

- In a large bowl, toss the sweet potato pieces with olive oil until evenly coated. Spread them out in a single layer on a baking sheet and bake for 20-25 minutes, or until tender and lightly browned.

- In a large saucepan or Dutch oven, sauté the onion and red bell pepper in a little bit of olive oil over medium heat until softened, about 5-7 minutes.

- Add the garlic, cumin, chili powder, paprika, and cayenne pepper to the saucepan, and cook for an additional 30 seconds, or until fragrant.

- Add the black beans, diced tomatoes (undrained), and vegetable broth to the saucepan. Stir everything together and bring to a simmer.

- Reduce the heat to low and let the chili simmer for 10-15 minutes, or until slightly thickened.

- Stir in the baked sweet potatoes and season with salt and pepper to taste.

- Serve hot, topped with chopped fresh cilantro, shredded cheese, sour cream or Greek yogurt if desired.

- This recipe makes about 4-6 servings, depending on your appetite. Each serving contains approximately 200-250 calories, 6-8g of protein, and 5-6g of fiber.

Chicken and vegetable fajitas with whole-wheat tortillas.

Ingredients:
1 lb boneless, skinless chicken breasts, sliced into thin strips
2 bell peppers (any color), sliced into thin strips
1 onion, sliced into thin strips
2 tablespoons olive oil
1 tablespoon chili powder
1 teaspoon cumin
1/2 teaspoon garlic powder
Salt and pepper to taste
8 whole-wheat tortillas

Optional toppings: sliced avocado, chopped cilantro, salsa, low-fat sour cream

Instructions:

- In a large bowl, combine the sliced chicken, bell peppers, onion, olive oil, chili powder, cumin, garlic powder, salt, and pepper. Toss everything together until the chicken and vegetables are evenly coated.

- Heat a large skillet over medium-high heat. Add the chicken and vegetable mixture and cook, stirring occasionally, for 8-10 minutes or until the chicken is cooked through and the vegetables are tender.

- Warm the tortillas in the microwave or in a dry skillet for a few seconds on each side.

- Serve the fajita mixture on the warm tortillas and top with sliced avocado, chopped cilantro, salsa, or low-fat sour cream if desired.

This recipe makes about 8 fajitas. Each fajita contains approximately 220-250 calories, 20-25g of protein, and 5-6g of fiber, depending on the size of the tortillas and the amount of toppings used.

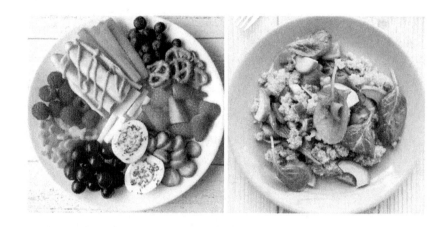

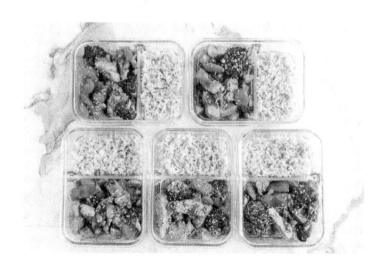

CHAPTER TWO

WEIGHT WATCHERS DIET DRINK RECIPES

Sparkling strawberry lemonade

Ingredients:

1/2 cup fresh strawberries, sliced

1/4 cup lemon juice

1/4 cup Truvia sweetener

3 cups sparkling water or club soda

Ice cubes

Fresh mint leaves (optional)

Directions:

- In a blender, puree the strawberries until smooth.

- In a pitcher, combine the strawberry puree, lemon juice, and Truvia sweetener.

- Stir until the sweetener is dissolved.

- Add the sparkling water or club soda to the pitcher and stir.

- Serve over ice cubes and garnish with fresh mint leaves (optional).

This recipe makes about 4 servings, with each serving containing approximately 10 calories and 0 Weight Watchers points. However, please note that the exact nutritional information may vary depending on the specific brands and amounts of ingredients used.

Iced green tea

Ingredients:
4 green tea bags
8 cups water
Ice cubes
Honey or lemon wedges for optional sweetening and flavoring

Directions:

- Boil 8 cups of water in a pot or kettle.

- Once the water has boiled, remove it from heat and add 4 green tea bags to the water.

- Steep the tea bags for 3-5 minutes, depending on your desired strength of tea.

- Remove the tea bags and let the tea cool to room temperature.

- Once the tea has cooled, pour it into a pitcher and refrigerate it for at least 30 minutes.

- When you're ready to serve, fill a glass with ice cubes and pour the iced green tea over the ice.

- Optionally, sweeten with honey or add a lemon wedge for flavor. Enjoy!

This recipe yields approximately 8 servings, depending on the size of the glasses used. Green tea is packed with antioxidants and other beneficial compounds, making it a healthy beverage option.

Pineapple smoothie

Ingredients:
2 cups fresh or frozen pineapple chunks
1 banana
1 cup coconut milk or almond milk
1/2 cup plain Greek yogurt
1 tbsp honey (optional)
Ice cubes (optional)

Directions:

- Add the pineapple chunks, banana, coconut milk or almond milk, and Greek yogurt to a blender.

- Blend on high speed until the mixture is smooth and creamy.

- Taste the smoothie and add honey if desired for extra sweetness.

- If the smoothie is too thick, add a few ice cubes to thin it out.

- Blend again until the ice cubes are crushed and well combined.

- Pour the smoothie into glasses and serve immediately.

- Enjoy!

This recipe makes about 2-3 servings depending on the size of the glasses used. Pineapple is a great source of vitamin C, while Greek yogurt provides protein and probiotics, making this smoothie a healthy and tasty snack or breakfast option.

Cucumber watermelon cooler

Ingredients:
2 cups diced watermelon
1/2 cup diced cucumber
1 lime, juiced
1-2 cups sparkling water or club soda
Ice cubes
Mint leaves for garnish (optional)

Directions:

- Add the diced watermelon, cucumber, and lime juice to a blender.

- Blend on high speed until the mixture is smooth and well combined.

- Pour the mixture into a pitcher.

- Add sparkling water or club soda to the pitcher, stirring well.

- Taste the mixture and adjust the sweetness and tanginess to your liking by adding more lime juice or a sweetener like honey or stevia.

- Add ice cubes to glasses and pour the cooler over the ice.

- Garnish with mint leaves if desired.

- Serve and enjoy!

This recipe makes about 2-3 servings, depending on the size of the glasses used. The watermelon adds sweetness and hydration, while the cucumber adds a refreshing and cooling effect, making this a perfect drink to cool down on a hot summer day.

Orange mango smoothie

Ingredients:

1 cup unsweetened almond milk

1 orange, peeled and segmented

1 cup frozen mango chunks

1 tablespoon chia seeds

1/2 teaspoon vanilla extract

1-2 teaspoons honey or agave syrup (optional)

Instructions:

- Add the almond milk to a blender.

- Add the orange segments, frozen mango chunks, chia seeds, vanilla extract, and honey or agave syrup (if using) to the blender.

- Blend on high until smooth and creamy, about 1-2 minutes.

- Taste and adjust the sweetness as needed.

- Pour into a glass and enjoy your Orange Mango smoothie!

This recipe makes one serving, but you can easily double or triple the ingredients to make more servings. The smoothie is low in calories, high in fiber, and packed with vitamins and antioxidants, making it a great option for weight watchers.

Berry blast smoothie

Ingredients:

1 cup frozen mixed berries (strawberries, raspberries, blackberries, blueberries)

1 banana, peeled

1/2 cup plain Greek yogurt

1/2 cup unsweetened almond milk

1 tablespoon honey or agave syrup

1/2 teaspoon vanilla extract

Optional: a handful of spinach or kale for extra nutrition

Instructions:

- Add the frozen mixed berries, banana, Greek yogurt, almond milk, honey or agave syrup, and vanilla extract to a blender.

- If desired, add a handful of spinach or kale to the blender for extra nutrition.

- Blend on high until smooth and creamy, about 1-2 minutes.

- Taste and adjust the sweetness as needed.

- Pour into a glass and enjoy your Berry Blast Smoothie!

This recipe makes one serving, but you can easily double or triple the ingredients to make more servings. The smoothie is high in fiber, protein, and antioxidants, making it a nutritious and satisfying meal or snack.

Minty cucumber limeade

Ingredients:
1 cucumber, peeled and chopped
1/2 cup fresh mint leaves
1/2 cup fresh lime juice (about 4-5 limes)
4 cups water
1-2 teaspoons honey or agave syrup (optional)
Ice cubes

Instructions:

- Add the chopped cucumber, mint leaves, and lime juice to a blender.

- Add water and honey or agave syrup (if using) to the blender.

- Blend on high until smooth and well combined, about 1-2 minutes.

- Taste and adjust the sweetness as needed.

- Pour the mixture through a fine mesh strainer into a pitcher.

- Serve over ice cubes and garnish with additional mint leaves and cucumber slices, if desired.

This recipe makes 4 servings. Each serving is low in calories and sugar, and high in vitamin C and antioxidants. It's a great way to stay hydrated and refreshed while following a weight watchers diet.

Watermelon lemonade

Ingredients:

4 cups cubed seedless watermelon

1/2 cup fresh lemon juice

4 cups cold water

1/4 cup honey or stevia (to taste)

Ice cubes

Lemon slices and mint leaves (optional garnish)

Instructions:

- In a blender, puree the watermelon until smooth.

- Strain the pureed watermelon through a fine-mesh sieve into a large pitcher to remove any pulp.

- Add the lemon juice, cold water, and honey or stevia to the pitcher and stir well until fully combined.

- Taste the lemonade and adjust sweetness as needed.

- Chill the lemonade in the refrigerator for at least 30 minutes before serving.

- Serve over ice and garnish with lemon slices and mint leaves if desired.

This watermelon lemonade recipe is low in calories and sugar, making it a perfect refreshing drink for weight watchers. Enjoy!

Spicy ginger lemonade

Ingredients:

1/2 cup fresh lemon juice

1/2 cup honey or stevia (to taste)

1/4 cup fresh ginger, peeled and grated

1/4 teaspoon cayenne pepper

4 cups cold water

Ice cubes

Lemon slices and fresh mint leaves (optional garnish)

Instructions:

- In a small saucepan, combine the honey or stevia, grated ginger, and cayenne pepper with 1/2 cup of water. Bring to a boil over medium heat, stirring constantly until the honey or stevia has dissolved.

- Remove from heat and let the mixture steep for 10-15 minutes to infuse the flavors of the ginger and cayenne pepper.

- Strain the ginger-cayenne mixture through a fine-mesh sieve into a large pitcher.

- Add the lemon juice and 4 cups of cold water to the pitcher, and stir well until fully combined.

- Taste the lemonade and adjust sweetness as needed.

- Chill the lemonade in the refrigerator for at least 30 minutes before serving.

- Serve over ice and garnish with lemon slices and fresh mint leaves if desired.

This spicy ginger lemonade is a low-calorie, low-sugar alternative to traditional lemonade, and the cayenne pepper provides a spicy kick that can help boost metabolism. Enjoy!

Apple cinnamon smoothie

Ingredients:
1 medium apple, peeled and chopped
1/2 cup plain Greek yogurt
1/2 cup unsweetened almond milk

1/2 teaspoon ground cinnamon

1 tablespoon honey or stevia (to taste)

Ice cubes (optional)

Instructions:

- Add the chopped apple, Greek yogurt, almond milk, cinnamon, and honey or stevia to a blender.

- If desired, add a few ice cubes to make the smoothie colder and thicker.

- Blend all ingredients until smooth and creamy.

- Taste the smoothie and adjust sweetness as needed.

- Pour into a glass and serve immediately.

This apple cinnamon smoothie is a healthy and filling breakfast or snack option that's packed with protein and fiber from the Greek yogurt and apple. Enjoy!

Blueberry lemonade

Ingredients:

1 cup fresh blueberries

1/2 cup fresh lemon juice

4 cups cold water

1/4 cup honey or stevia (to taste)

Ice cubes

Lemon slices and fresh mint leaves (optional garnish)

Instructions:

- In a blender, puree the blueberries until smooth.

- Strain the pureed blueberries through a fine-mesh sieve into a large pitcher to remove any pulp.

- Add the lemon juice, cold water, and honey or stevia to the pitcher and stir well until fully combined.

- Taste the lemonade and adjust sweetness as needed.

- Chill the lemonade in the refrigerator for at least 30 minutes before serving.

- Serve over ice and garnish with lemon slices and fresh mint leaves if desired.

This blueberry lemonade recipe is low in calories and sugar, making it a perfect refreshing drink for weight watchers. The blueberries add a boost of antioxidants and vitamins to the lemonade. Enjoy!

Peach iced tea

Ingredients:

4 cups water

4 black tea bags

2 ripe peaches, peeled and sliced

1/4 cup honey or stevia (to taste)

Ice cubes

Peach slices and fresh mint leaves (optional garnish)

Instructions:

- In a large pot, bring the water to a boil.

- Add the black tea bags and steep for 3-5 minutes until the tea is strong.

- Remove the tea bags and add the sliced peaches to the pot.

- Reduce the heat to low and let the peaches simmer for 5-10 minutes until they are soft and the tea is infused with peach flavor.

- Remove the pot from the heat and let it cool for 10-15 minutes.

- Strain the tea and peaches through a fine-mesh sieve into a large pitcher.

- Add the honey or stevia to the pitcher and stir well until fully combined.

- Chill the tea in the refrigerator for at least 30 minutes before serving.

- Serve over ice and garnish with peach slices and fresh mint leaves if desired.

This peach iced tea recipe is a low-calorie and low-sugar alternative to traditional sweet tea. The peaches add natural sweetness and flavor to the tea, and the honey or stevia provides just the right amount of sweetness. Enjoy!

Pineapple mint mojito

Ingredients:

1 cup fresh pineapple chunks
1/4 cup fresh mint leaves
1/4 cup lime juice
1/4 cup honey or stevia (to taste)
1/4 cup white rum
Club soda
Ice cubes
Pineapple wedges and fresh mint leaves (optional garnish)

Instructions:

- In a blender, puree the pineapple chunks and mint leaves until smooth.

- Strain the pureed mixture through a fine-mesh sieve into a large pitcher.

- Add the lime juice, honey or stevia, and white rum to the pitcher and stir well until fully combined.

- Fill a glass with ice cubes and pour the pineapple mint mixture over the ice.

- Top the glass off with club soda and stir gently

- Taste the mojito and adjust sweetness or lime juice as needed.

- Garnish with pineapple wedges and fresh mint leaves if desired.

This Pineapple Mint Mojito is a refreshing and tropical drink that's perfect for a summer day or a special occasion. The combination of pineapple, mint, and lime creates a flavorful and balanced cocktail, and the use of honey or stevia instead of sugar makes it a healthier option. Enjoy!

Iced vanilla latte

Ingredients:

1 shot of espresso

1 cup unsweetened vanilla almond milk (or any other non-dairy milk of your choice)

1 tsp vanilla extract

1 tsp honey (optional)

Ice cubes

Instructions:

- Brew a shot of espresso using an espresso machine or stovetop espresso maker.

- Add the vanilla extract and honey (if using) to the espresso and stir to combine.

- Pour the unsweetened vanilla almond milk into a glass and add ice cubes.

- Pour the espresso mixture over the ice and stir to combine.

- Enjoy your Iced Vanilla Latte!

Weight Watchers Points:

Espresso shot: 0 points

Unsweetened vanilla almond milk: 1 point

Honey (1 tsp): 1 point

Total: 2 points

Note: You can adjust the amount of honey or omit it altogether to suit your taste preferences and Weight Watchers points budget.

Raspberry lemonade

Ingredients:

1 cup fresh raspberries

1/2 cup freshly squeezed lemon juice (about 3 lemons)

4 cups cold water

1/4 cup honey (or more to taste)

Ice cubes

Fresh mint leaves (optional)

Instructions:

- In a blender or food processor, puree the raspberries until smooth.

- In a large pitcher, combine the raspberry puree, lemon juice, water, and honey. Stir well to combine.

- Taste and adjust the sweetness as needed.

- Chill in the refrigerator for at least 1 hour.

- When ready to serve, add ice cubes and fresh mint leaves (if using) to the pitcher.

- Stir well and pour into individual glasses. Enjoy your Raspberry Lemonade!

Weight Watchers Points:
Raspberries: 0 points
Lemon juice: 0 points
Honey (1/4 cup): 12 points
Total: 12 points

Note: You can adjust the amount of honey or omit it altogether to suit your taste preferences and Weight Watchers points budget. You can also use a sugar substitute like Stevia to reduce the points.

Grapefruit and ginger spritzer

Ingredients:
2 cups fresh grapefruit juice (about 2 grapefruits)
1/4 cup freshly grated ginger
4 cups sparkling water
1/4 cup honey (or more to taste)
Ice cubes
Fresh rosemary sprigs (optional)

Instructions:

- In a large pitcher, combine the grapefruit juice, grated ginger, sparkling water, and honey. Stir well to combine.

- Taste and adjust the sweetness as needed.

- Chill in the refrigerator for at least 1 hour.

- When ready to serve, add ice cubes and fresh rosemary sprigs (if using) to the pitcher.

- Stir well and pour into individual glasses.

- Enjoy your Grapefruit and Ginger Spritzer!

Weight Watchers Points:
Grapefruit juice: 0 points
Ginger: 0 points
Honey (1/4 cup): 12 points
Sparkling water: 0 points
Total: 12 points

Note: You can adjust the amount of honey or omit it altogether to suit your taste preferences and Weight Watchers points budget. You can also use a sugar substitute like Stevia to reduce the points.

Chocolate banana smoothie

Ingredients:

1 ripe banana

1 cup unsweetened vanilla almond milk (or any other non-dairy milk of your choice)

1 tbsp unsweetened cocoa powder

1/2 tsp vanilla extract

1 tsp honey (optional)

Ice cubes

Instructions:

- Peel the banana and cut it into chunks.

- In a blender, combine the banana chunks, unsweetened vanilla almond milk, unsweetened cocoa powder, vanilla extract, and honey (if using).

- Blend until smooth and creamy.

- Add ice cubes to the blender and blend again until the smoothie is thick and frosty.

- Pour into a glass and serve immediately.

- Enjoy your Chocolate Banana Smoothie!

Weight Watchers Points:

Banana: 0 points

Unsweetened vanilla almond milk: 1 point

Unsweetened cocoa powder: 0 points

Honey (1 tsp): 1 point

Total: 2 points

Note: You can adjust the amount of honey or omit it altogether to suit your taste preferences and Weight Watchers points budget. You can also add a scoop of protein powder or a tablespoon of nut butter to increase the protein and healthy fat content.

Mango iced tea

Ingredients:

2 mangoes, peeled and chopped

4 cups water

4 tea bags (black tea or green tea)

1/4 cup honey

Ice cubes

Instructions:

- In a blender, puree the chopped mangoes until smooth.

- In a medium-sized saucepan, bring 4 cups of water to a boil.

- Add the tea bags to the boiling water and let it steep for 5-10 minutes, depending on the strength of tea you prefer.

- Remove the tea bags and let the tea cool down to room temperature.

- Once the tea has cooled down, stir in the honey until it dissolves.

- Add the mango puree to the tea and stir well.

- Chill the mixture in the refrigerator for a couple of hours until it is completely cold.

- Serve the Mango Iced Tea in glasses filled with ice cubes.

This recipe makes around 4 servings, and each serving contains around 70-80 calories, which is suitable for a weight watchers diet. However, it's important to keep in mind that this drink does contain natural sugars from the mangoes and honey, so it should be consumed in moderation as part of a balanced diet.

Pomegranate iced tea

Ingredients:
4 cups water
4 tea bags (black tea or green tea)
1/2 cup pomegranate juice

1/4 cup honey

Ice cubes

Pomegranate seeds (optional)

Instructions:

- In a medium-sized saucepan, bring 4 cups of water to a boil.

- Add the tea bags to the boiling water and let it steep for 5-10 minutes, depending on the strength of tea you prefer.

- Remove the tea bags and let the tea cool down to room temperature.

- Once the tea has cooled down, stir in the pomegranate juice and honey until they dissolve.

- Chill the mixture in the refrigerator for a couple of hours until it is completely cold.

- Serve the Pomegranate Iced Tea in glasses filled with ice cubes.

- Garnish with pomegranate seeds if desired.

This recipe makes around 4 servings, and each serving contains around 70-80 calories, which is suitable for a weight watchers diet. The pomegranate juice adds a refreshing twist to traditional iced tea and is a good source of antioxidants. However, it's important to keep in mind that this drink does contain natural sugars from the pomegranate juice and honey, so it should be consumed in moderation as part of a balanced diet.

Turmeric ginger lemonade

Ingredients:

4 cups water

1/4 cup fresh turmeric root, peeled and grated

1/4 cup fresh ginger root, peeled and grated

1/2 cup freshly squeezed lemon juice

1/4 cup honey

Ice cubes

Lemon slices and fresh mint leaves (optional)

Instructions:

- In a medium-sized saucepan, bring 4 cups of water to a boil.

- Add the grated turmeric and ginger to the boiling water and let it simmer for 5-10 minutes.

- Remove the saucepan from the heat and let the mixture cool down to room temperature.

- Once the mixture has cooled down, strain it through a fine-mesh sieve or cheesecloth to remove the solids.

- Stir in the freshly squeezed lemon juice and honey until they dissolve.

- Chill the mixture in the refrigerator for a couple of hours until it is completely cold.

- Serve the Turmeric Ginger Lemonade in glasses filled with ice cubes.

- Garnish with lemon slices and fresh mint leaves if desired.

This recipe makes around 4 servings, and each serving contains around 60-70 calories, which is suitable for a weight watchers diet. Turmeric and ginger have anti-inflammatory properties, while lemon provides a good source of vitamin C. However, it's important to keep in mind that honey is a natural sweetener and does contain calories, so it should be used in moderation as part of a balanced diet.

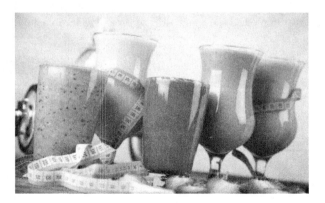

AUTHOR ADVICE

I'd be happy to help! Here are some tips for someone who wants to use the Weight Watchers Diet Book in 2023:

Understand the basics: Weight Watchers works on a points system, where each food is assigned a certain number of points based on its nutritional value. You are assigned a certain number of daily points based on your weight and goals, and you track your points throughout the day.

Plan your meals: Take some time to plan out your meals for the week ahead of time. This can help you stay on track and make sure you're getting a good balance of nutrients.

Be mindful of portion sizes: Even healthy foods can be high in calories, so it's important to pay attention to portion sizes. Use measuring cups and a food scale to ensure you're not overeating.

Make healthy swaps: Look for ways to make your favorite meals healthier. For example, you could swap out white rice for brown rice, or use Greek yogurt instead of sour cream.

Keep healthy snacks on hand: It's important to have healthy snacks available for when you get hungry between meals. Some good options include fresh fruit, vegetables, nuts, and low-fat cheese.

Drink plenty of water: Drinking water can help you feel full and satisfied, and it's important for overall health. Aim to drink at least 8 glasses of water per day.

Be patient: Weight loss is a gradual process, and it's important to be patient and stick with your plan even if you don't see immediate results. Celebrate small victories along the way, and remember that slow and steady progress is more sustainable than rapid weight loss.

Track your progress: Use the tracking tools in the Weight Watchers Diet Book to monitor your progress over time. This can help you identify areas where you're doing well and areas where you might need to make adjustments.

Allow for flexibility: While it's important to stick to your daily points target as closely as possible, it's also important to allow for some flexibility. If you have a special occasion or social event, for example, you might need to use some of your weekly points to enjoy a treat or two.

Try new recipes: The Weight Watchers Diet Book includes a variety of recipes that are healthy and delicious. Trying new recipes can help keep things interesting and prevent boredom.

Don't skip meals: Skipping meals can actually make it harder to lose weight. Make sure you're eating enough throughout the day to keep your energy levels up and avoid overeating later on.

Find healthy ways to cope with stress: Stress can often trigger unhealthy eating habits. Finding healthy ways to cope with stress, such as exercise or meditation, can help you stay on track.

Stay accountable: It's important to stay accountable to yourself and your goals. You can do this by tracking your progress, sharing your goals with others, or joining a Weight Watchers group.

Celebrate your successes: Celebrating your successes, no matter how small, can help keep you motivated and on track. Whether it's treating yourself to a new outfit or sharing your success with a friend, take the time to acknowledge your hard work and achievements.

Remember, the Weight Watchers Diet Book is just a tool to help you achieve your weight loss goals. It's up to you to make healthy choices and commit to a healthy lifestyle over the long term. With dedication, patience, and support, you can achieve your goals and live a happier, healthier life.

Printed in Great Britain
by Amazon

23139763R00046